Dangerous Pussi

Owning Your Feminine Fire After a Hysterectomy

Written By
Icy Kendrick

ICY KENDRICK

Dangerous Pussi : Owning your Feminine Fire After A Hysterectomy

To every woman who has walked through fire to find herself whole on the other side this is for you. To the ones who have redefined what it means to be powerful, to be feminine, to be complete. May this book be a reminder that you are so much more than what the world sees or defines you by. Here's to your courage, your grace, and your fierce, unyielding spirit.

And to my family, who has stood by me through every twist, every turn, and every step of becoming: thank you for being my Strength.

– Icy

"In the strength of surrender, I found the deepest power. In the softness of acceptance, I discovered resilience. And in letting go of what no longer served me, I reclaimed everything I truly am."

- Icy Kendrick

Contents

Foreword

Sacred Rituals to Honor the Energy of Your Womb Space

Honoring your womb space is a powerful way to reconnect with your inner self and reclaim your feminine energy. These sacred rituals are designed to help you tap into the wisdom that lives within you, to celebrate the cycles of your life, and to hold space for all that you are.

1. The Candle of Creation Ritual

- **Purpose**: This ritual is for honoring the creative energy of your womb space, a place of ideas, dreams, and passions.

- **How to Practice**: Light a candle and place it on a small altar or sacred space. Sit in front of the flame, close your eyes, and place your hands over your lower abdomen. As you breathe deeply, visualize a golden light radiating from your womb space, connecting with the flame. This light represents your creativity, your strength, and the energy that flows within you. Reflect on the ways in which you are a creator in your life—whether through nurturing others, building dreams, or bringing love into the world. Allow this ritual to remind you that your womb space is a sacred source of creation, regardless of physical form.

2. Moonlight Cleansing

- **Purpose**: To cleanse and refresh the energy of your womb space, letting go of old emotions or pain and inviting healing and renewal.

- **How to Practice**: On a night when the moon is bright, stand outside or by a window where you can feel its light. Place one hand on your heart and the other over your lower belly. Breathe in deeply, imagining the moonlight washing over you, filling your womb space with calm, healing energy. Visualize any heaviness, sorrow, or lingering energy releasing from your body, leaving you light and renewed. This ritual can be especially meaningful during the full moon, a time for release and transformation.

3. The Rose Ceremony

- **Purpose**: To honor the softness and strength of your womb space and your feminine spirit.

- **How to Practice**: Select a fresh rose, symbolizing beauty, resilience, and love. Sit in a quiet space with the rose, breathing deeply. Gently hold the rose over your womb space and speak words of love and appreciation for yourself. Reflect on your journey, acknowledging the beauty and wisdom within. When you're ready, place the rose petals in a bowl of water. This bowl can be kept on your altar or in a place where you'll see it as a reminder of your strength and grace.

Womb Honoring Ceremony

This ceremony is an act of reverence, a way to honor the spirit of your womb, whether it is physically present or not. It is a reminder that the womb space lives within you as a source of wisdom, intuition, and creation.

Create a Sacred Space: Find a quiet place and surround yourself with things that bring you peace candles, crystals, flowers, or meaningful objects. Play soft music if it helps you connect with the moment.

Grounding Breath: Sit or lie comfortably and take several deep, grounding breaths. Place one hand on your heart and the other over your womb space. Feel the connection between these two centers, the warmth and the energy flowing between them.

Speak Words of Honor: Out loud or in your mind, speak to your womb space with love and gratitude. Say something like:

"Thank you for holding my stories, my dreams, my resilience."

"I honor the wisdom you carry, the strength you hold, and the spirit of creation within you."

"I release any sorrow, guilt, or pain that may linger here, and I welcome healing, love, and peace."

Blessing with Water: Dip your fingers in a small bowl of water, blessing it with intentions of healing and empowerment. Gently touch this water to your womb space, imagining it as a balm, soothing and nourishing you.

Seal with a Symbol: End the ceremony by drawing a symbol of strength over your womb space this could be a heart, a spiral, or any symbol that resonates with you. Let this be a sign of your commitment to honor yourself fully, to cherish your feminine spirit, and to hold your womb space as sacred.

Inspiring Words of Strength

To my sisters who walk this journey of honoring their womb space, remember: You are whole, complete, and powerful. You are not defined by what you have or have not lost. You are defined by the strength, resilience, and love that lives within you. Your womb space is a vessel of energy, creativity, and wisdom, no matter its physical form. Embrace it, honor it, and allow it to guide you.

In times of doubt, let your hands rest over your womb, and remember that you carry within you the stories of generations, the strength of all who came before you. Trust in your power, in your journey, and in the beauty of your rebirth. You are a woman of infinite grace, unwavering courage, and boundless love. Stand in this truth, and let it light the path ahead.

May these sacred stories, rituals, and this ceremony remind you that your womb space is an eternal source of wisdom and strength, a place that holds your essence beyond form or structure. Embrace this sacred journey of honoring your womb space, knowing that you are connected to a powerful lineage of women who, like you, carry the sacred within.

Preface

Preface: Sacred Stories of Womb History and Rituals to Honor Your Womb Space

Our wombs carry stories deep, ancient histories of resilience, creation, transformation, and wisdom. Even when our physical wombs change or no longer reside within us, the energy of that sacred space remains, a vibrant center of power and intuition. The womb, in all its symbolism, holds our experiences and those of countless women who came before us. To honor our womb space is to honor our lineage, our feminine energy, and the cycles of life and rebirth within ourselves.

The stories of our wombs are not merely biological they are spiritual, emotional, and soulful. They hold the memories of life's ebbs and flows, of love given and received, of strength forged through both joy and hardship. Every woman who has felt the ache of change in her womb or who has learned to let go of the physical womb while embracing its energy knows this truth: the power of the womb is unbreakable. It lives within us, guiding and grounding us, reminding us that we are more than the sum of our parts.

This preface is dedicated to the rituals and ceremonies that help us reconnect with and honor this powerful space within us, to remember that we are part of a lineage that stretches across generations. Let these practices be an invitation to hold your womb space with reverence, no matter your physical state, and to recognize that your feminine energy is whole, complete, and radiant, exactly as it is.

Introduction

Introduction: The Journey to Reclaiming Power

When I think about femininity and power, it's a journey that's taken on many faces in my life. For so long, these words seemed like defined, unchanging things, set out by expectations and norms that never quite fit. But the truth is, they're anything but static. For those of us who've had to confront a part of ourselves being taken, altered, or changed beyond recognition especially through something as life-altering as a hysterectomy femininity and power become concepts we get to redefine, and ultimately, reclaim.

This journey is not just about what has been lost, but about what's waiting to be discovered. So much of our culture attaches femininity to physical attributes, like the womb. We're led to believe that our power as women stems from the potential to give life, to nurture, and to be whole in one very specific way. But what if we are whole without any conditions, without any attachments to what society tells us we must be?

I wrote this book because I know what it feels like to wonder who you are on the other side of profound change. For anyone who's felt that same pull, that same ache to understand herself in new ways, this book is here to guide you through your own rediscovery. This journey isn't about fitting back into a box, but about throwing that box away entirely and seeing what feminine power truly means when it's just about *you*.

I invite you to embrace your resilience and tap into that deep, untamed part of yourself. Together, we're stepping into a version of femininity that's not defined by anyone else's rules. Here, power is what you say it is. Femininity is whatever feels right and true to you. Let this be your companion through every reflection, every realization, and every step you take toward reclaiming your true, powerful, feminine self.

1

Chapter 1: The Girl Who Thought She Knew It All

Growing up, I was the girl who thought she had it all figured out. In my mind, I wasn't just a regular kid I was wise beyond my years, or so I thought. I remember sitting under the Elders, absorbing every word they spoke, believing that by listening closely, I was gaining the kind of wisdom only they could give. Their stories, insights, and teachings made me feel special, as though I was receiving a secret knowledge that set me apart from everyone else my age. I thought, *If I just listen enough, if I understand enough, I'll have all the answers.*

And at twelve years old, that was exactly what I believed: that I knew it all. In my heart, I thought I could see every angle, understand every outcome, and avoid every mistake. I felt as though I was being given a map to life, and with it, I could avoid the rough terrain and skip straight to smooth sailing. But here's the thing the journey of life doesn't work that way. Sitting with the Elders gave me knowledge, yes, but it wasn't the same as living my own story.

There's a profound difference between *knowing* the journey and *living* the journey. Knowing is safe; it's comfortable and full of certainties. But living? Living means getting bruised, taking wrong turns, and facing detours that make you question every bit of knowledge you thought you had. I learned that the hard way as I grew older, as I started living experiences that no amount of wisdom from others could fully prepare me for.

The Elders taught me so much, but their wisdom was only a foundation it couldn't be the whole story. I had to learn to respect that, even if I felt wise or well-prepared, life would always have more lessons to teach me. And those lessons wouldn't always be gentle or come in the form of quiet advice. Sometimes, they would come crashing into my world, challenging everything I thought I knew.

Looking back, I can see that my younger self wasn't wrong for wanting answers. She wasn't foolish for seeking shortcuts or believing she could skip the messier parts of life. She was simply young, full of hope, and eager to find a way to feel in control. But control is an illusion we only hold onto when we haven't yet lived through the unpredictability of real life.

As I grew older, I had to honor the wisdom of that girl who thought she knew it all, while also learning to let go of her need to *know everything.* There is wisdom we all hold within us, yes, but that wisdom is a seed it needs the experiences of life to grow into something more. Life has a way of humbling us, of showing us that true wisdom is less about having answers and more about being open to the questions.

This chapter is a reminder that, no matter how wise we think we are, life will always have new lessons in store. We are never finished learning, never complete in our understanding. True power comes from respecting that journey, from knowing that while we may hold wisdom, we're also students of life. And that, ultimately, is where our greatest strength lies.

2

Chapter 2: The Mirror of Reality and the Masks We Wear

From the moment we open our eyes to the world, we're surrounded by reflections. Our family, our friends, our culture everything around us shapes the person we come to believe we are. It's as if every interaction, every word, and every belief we take in creates a mirror, one that shows us not just our face, but what we start to think is our truth. And without realizing it, we begin to wear masks shaped by those reflections, allowing our surroundings to define us before we even have a chance to decide who we truly want to be.

In those early years, when our identities are still forming, we're incredibly impressionable. We're like sponges, absorbing the beliefs and behaviors of everyone around us. If we're told we're smart, we start to believe it; if we're told we're not enough, that too becomes part of our self-image. We reflect what we see and hear, and in many ways, we mirror the world around us. But the danger in this is that those reflections often come from others' projections, limitations, and unresolved wounds. It can be difficult to separate what's truly ours from what we've merely picked up along the way.

This is where the masks begin to form. We put them on without realizing, adapting to the expectations and judgments of others, hoping to fit into the mold that has been created for us. These masks serve a purpose, protecting us from judgment or rejection, helping us navigate a world that can feel overwhelmingly confining. But in time, these masks become a trap. We start to believe that the face we present to the world is the only face we have, forgetting that there's a deeper self hidden beneath it all.

For many of us, the weight of wearing these masks becomes too heavy. We feel "boxed in" by a reality that doesn't quite fit, but we don't know how to break free. This is where escapism comes in—a way to loosen the grip of those masks, to momentarily feel lighter, freer, unbound by the expectations of others. Whether it's through daydreaming, indulging in fantasy, or seeking solace in people or substances, escapism can feel like a lifeline when reality feels too tight. It offers us a moment of release, a glimpse of who we might be if we could just tear those masks away.

But escapism, as comforting as it might be in the moment, is only temporary. It doesn't take away the mask; it only lets us forget it for a while. When we return, the reality remains, and so do the masks. Worse yet, the longer we wear them, the harder it becomes to distinguish between who we really are and who we're pretending to be. Escapism becomes less about freedom and more about avoiding the discomfort of facing the real work of discovering our authentic selves.

One of the most profound lessons I've learned is that our self-perception can be deeply distorted by these social mirrors and the masks they create. The way we see ourselves often reflects not who we truly are, but the judgments and limitations that others have placed upon us. Our self-worth becomes entangled with these reflections, and we begin to believe that we are only as valuable as others perceive us to be. It's as if we've handed over the power to define ourselves to everyone around us, never realizing that this power was ours all along.

To break free from this cycle, we have to look beyond the mirror of reality and strip away the masks we wear. We have to question the beliefs we've internalized, asking ourselves: *Is this really mine? Does this belief serve me, or does it hold me back?* We have to be brave enough to face our true reflection, even if it's unfamiliar, even if it challenges everything we thought we knew about ourselves.

This chapter is an invitation to let go of the masks and step away from the mirrors that have distorted our self-image. It's a call to reclaim our power to define who we are, independent of the expectations and judgments of others. Because true self-worth isn't found in the reflections of others it's discovered in the quiet, unmasked moments when we finally see ourselves as we are, and love what we see.

3

Chapter 3: Escapism vs. Empowerment

Escapism is one of those things we all reach for when life feels too heavy, too complicated, or simply too much to bear. It's an action, a choice we make, consciously or not, to put life on pause and step outside of our reality, even if just for a moment. In that instant, escapism promises us relief from whatever weighs us down. It's the deep sigh we exhale when we shut out the world, the sense of freedom that comes when we lose ourselves in fantasy or distraction. But for many of us, escapism has become more than an occasional relief it's become a coping mechanism, a way to avoid facing the things we fear the most.

For women, especially those navigating bodily changes, escapism can hold a powerful allure. In a society that often defines us by our physical form, any change—particularly those that affect our sense of femininity can feel overwhelming. We feel the eyes of the world watching us, assessing our worth based on standards we never agreed to, and that scrutiny can be crushing. When our bodies change, we may struggle to recognize ourselves, to accept this new reality that doesn't fit neatly into the world's expectations. And so, we look for ways to escape, to silence the inner dialogue that questions our worth and avoid the reality that feels too raw, too personal, to confront head-on.

But what happens when there's nowhere left to run? There comes a point when the act of escaping no longer brings the peace we seek. We can avoid, deny, and distract ourselves, but eventually, life brings us to a moment of truth—a place where there are no more hiding spots, no more ways to delay facing what's within. We stand at a crossroads, where the choice becomes clear: keep running or turn and face ourselves, masks off, in all our vulnerable, unguarded truth.

This is where empowerment begins. Empowerment isn't about living a life free from challenges or pain; it's about finding the courage to stand still in the face of those things and embrace who we are within them. To be empowered is to channel the energy we once used for escapism into something purposeful, something that connects us to ourselves instead of disconnecting us from reality. Empowerment is a choice, an active decision to stay present, to explore, and to heal.

Choosing to channel rather than escape is an act of defiance against a world that often tells us to bury our pain and carry on. When we choose to channel, we're saying, *I will not run from myself. I will meet my truth with open arms.* Channeling is about taking the intensity of our experiences, the depth of our emotions, and using them to fuel something transformative. It's a way to take our pain and turn it into art, movement, or insight.

Channeling is about using every part of our story the beautiful, the broken, and the raw to build a life that feels authentic and meaningful.

Standing face to face with ourselves without a mask is not easy. It requires us to sit with emotions we may have avoided for years, to confront fears we've kept hidden, and to challenge beliefs we've held onto simply because they felt safe. But in this process, we discover a power we never knew we had the power to shape our lives from a place of authenticity, to make choices that honor who we are and where we want to go.

Escapism may offer temporary comfort, but empowerment offers lasting peace. Empowerment allows us to live fully, to engage with life's challenges as they come, and to know that we have the strength to meet them head-on. When we channel rather than escape, we reclaim the parts of ourselves that we once abandoned, and in doing so, we become whole. We no longer see our challenges as things to avoid but as opportunities to grow and redefine what power means to us.

This chapter is an invitation to let go of escapism and embrace empowerment. It's a call to channel your energy, to stand in your truth, and to use your journey as fuel for something greater. Because the real power lies not in running from ourselves but in having the courage to stay, to grow, and to thrive right where we are.

4

Chapter 4: The Art of Surrendering to Growth

In the Tarot, the Hanged Man hangs suspended, upside-down, caught in a moment of complete surrender. For some, this card may seem unsettling at first glance, symbolizing a kind of forced stillness. But look closer, and you'll see that the Hanged Man isn't struggling or resisting. He is calm, almost serene, as though he has come to accept his position. This archetype teaches us something profound about the nature of surrender and growth that sometimes, to truly transform, we must first let go and allow life to take us in a new direction, even if that direction feels uncomfortable or unexpected.

The Hanged Man represents those moments when the universe itself seems to halt us in our tracks, setting us in a position that demands patience, reflection, and, above all, surrender. Often, these moments aren't ones we would choose they may come in the form of challenges, unexpected changes, or losses that shift our world. But the beauty of the Hanged Man is that he shows us the power in releasing control, in choosing to embrace what is rather than fighting against it.

For so many of us, surrender feels like defeat. We are taught to push forward, to stay in control, to hold on tightly to the path we envisioned. But the art of surrendering to growth is not about giving up; it's about recognizing that sometimes, life has a wisdom beyond our understanding. When we release our grip and allow ourselves to be held by life's current, we open up space for transformation that goes deeper than we could ever have planned. Surrendering to growth means choosing to believe that the universe is guiding us, placing us in the exact situations we need to become the person we are meant to be.

There is a quiet strength in surrender. It takes courage to let go of the desire to control every outcome and to trust that even in our most challenging times, there is a purpose unfolding. This surrender doesn't mean we are passive or that we give up on our dreams; rather, it means that we are willing to adjust, to accept, and to grow in response to life's unpredictable nature. This willingness to flow, to shift, and to remain open is one of the purest forms of maturity and true feminine power.

I have learned from wise women that maturity isn't about having all the answers or always knowing the right path. True maturity, they taught me, is about having the humility to accept what we cannot control and the strength to adapt to the circumstances life gives us. These women showed me that feminine power is rooted not in unyielding strength but in graceful resilience. They taught me that surrendering to growth is about understanding that each twist and turn, each pause and setback, is an invitation to learn and expand.

To surrender to growth is to embody the grace of the feminine spirit. It is a commitment to trust life, to lean into discomfort, and to believe that our experiences no matter how difficult are shaping us into the women we are meant to become. This doesn't mean we ignore our pain or pretend that challenges are easy; instead, we honor our struggles, recognizing them as sacred parts of our journey. We allow ourselves to feel, to grieve, and to process, knowing that this openness is the very thing that allows us to transform.

The art of surrender is an act of faith, a decision to believe that life's design holds more wisdom than our own limited vision. It is in surrendering that we find true power, not in the resistance or the struggle, but in the softening, the acceptance, and the willingness to embrace whatever comes. This chapter is an invitation to let go, to release the need to control, and to trust that life has your best interests at heart. Growth is rarely comfortable, but it is always sacred.

In the quiet space of surrender, we find ourselves, stripped of our illusions and closer to our essence. This is the essence of feminine power the strength to surrender, the grace to grow, and the courage to trust in life's journey, wherever it may lead.

5

Chapter 5: Redefining Femininity Without Wombs

For many of us, society has long defined femininity in narrow, biologically driven terms, tying womanhood to the ability to give life, nurture, and embody certain physical characteristics. But femininity is so much more than biology. After a hysterectomy, many women face a deeply personal question: *What does femininity mean to me now?* This chapter is about finding your own answer, about expanding your sense of self beyond society's expectations and myths to redefine femininity as something that lives in your spirit, your creativity, and your unique essence.

Addressing Myths and Misconceptions About Femininity Post-Hysterectomy

The world is filled with myths about what it means to be a woman, and many of these myths are rooted in outdated beliefs. One of the most common misconceptions is that a woman's worth or femininity is directly tied to her ability to have children. But femininity is far richer and more complex than this narrow definition.

A hysterectomy doesn't make anyone less of a woman, nor does it take away the feminine essence that lives within us. Femininity is not defined by physical organs it's an energy, an expression, a way of moving through the world with grace, creativity, intuition, and strength. This chapter invites you to dismantle these myths and release any guilt, shame, or confusion you may feel around what it means to be a woman post–hysterectomy.

Reclaiming Femininity as Energy, Creativity, and Essence

True femininity is about so much more than biology. It's an energy, a life force that exists within each of us, flowing through our creativity, compassion, and strength. This feminine essence is about embracing who we are, feeling deeply, and living authentically. When we redefine femininity as an energy, we free ourselves from limiting beliefs and open up to a broader, more inclusive understanding of what it means to be a woman.

Femininity is also deeply connected to our creativity. This doesn't necessarily mean artistic talents it's about the power to create in all aspects of life. It's the way we nurture relationships, grow ideas, and bring beauty into the world around us. Whether it's through art, work, or acts of kindness, this creativity is an essential part of feminine energy.

And finally, femininity is a state of being. It's the confidence we carry, the wisdom we share, and the love we give. It's about connecting with our true selves, honoring our intuition, and knowing that our value isn't based on what we can or cannot do, but simply on who we are. When we redefine femininity as energy, creativity, and essence, we reclaim it as something personal, powerful, and uniquely ours.

Embracing a New Feminine Identity Through Spiritual and Personal Growth

Redefining femininity often requires us to look inward and embark on a journey of spiritual and personal growth. This process is about finding a new connection to ourselves, a new understanding of who we are outside of physical definitions. It's an invitation to explore what femininity means to us individually, independent of any labels or limitations.

Connect with Your Spiritual Essence: Whether through meditation, prayer, or quiet reflection, spend time reconnecting with your inner self. Ask yourself: *What does being feminine mean to me now?* Listen for the answers that come from within, allowing your own spirit to guide you.

Create Rituals for Self-Care and Reflection: Femininity is deeply rooted in self-love and nurturing. Develop rituals that help you care for yourself emotionally, mentally, and physically. This could be as simple as setting aside time each week for self-reflection, taking a bath, journaling, or lighting a candle to symbolize your commitment to yourself.

Explore Feminine Archetypes: Many spiritual traditions honor feminine archetypes, such as the Warrior, the Nurturer, the Sage, and the Lover. Explore these archetypes and see which resonate with you as expressions of your own femininity. This can help you find new ways to relate to and celebrate the multifaceted nature of being a woman.

Embrace Your Intuition: Intuition is often associated with feminine wisdom, a deep inner knowing that guides us. Practice listening to your intuition, allowing it to lead you in making decisions and understanding yourself more deeply. This is a powerful way to connect with your feminine energy, one that is grounded in trust and self-awareness.

Exercises to Reconnect with Your Inner Feminine Power and Redefine Your Story

Reclaiming femininity post-hysterectomy is a journey of reconnection. Here are some exercises to help you tap into your inner feminine power, redefine your story, and embrace a new sense of self.

Writing Your Own Definition of Femininity

- Take a few minutes to reflect on what femininity means to you. Write down your own definition one that feels empowering, authentic, and aligned with who you are now.

- Reflect on questions like: *How do I express my femininity? What qualities do I admire in myself and other women? What aspects of my personality feel feminine to me?*
- Revisit this definition often, adding to it as you continue to grow and redefine your sense of self.

2. Mirror Work for Self-Embrace

- Stand in front of a mirror and look at yourself with kindness and love. Speak affirmations like: *I am powerful, I am feminine, I am enough just as I am.*

- This exercise may feel challenging at first, but mirror work can be incredibly healing. It allows you to see yourself as you are and embrace your beauty and femininity, free of judgment or comparison.

3. Creative Expression as a Channel for Feminine Energy

- Pick a creative activity that resonates with you drawing, painting, dancing, writing poetry, or even cooking. Dedicate time to this activity, allowing yourself to create without rules or restrictions.

- Let this be a space for you to express your emotions, dreams, and inner world. Embrace the process as an act of honoring your feminine power, reconnecting with your unique voice and creativity.

4. **Connecting with Nature as a Source of Feminine Wisdom**

- Spend time in nature, observing its cycles, rhythms, and beauty. Notice how nature embodies the essence of femininity: growth, creation, transformation, and balance.

- Nature reminds us that we are part of a larger, natural cycle, and that our bodies and spirits hold wisdom that goes beyond cultural definitions. Use this connection to reaffirm your own strength, resilience, and beauty.

5. **Meditation for Reclaiming Feminine Power**

- Sit quietly, breathing deeply, and focus on a part of your body that feels powerful or comforting to you. This could be your heart, your hands, or any part that feels aligned with your sense of self.

- Visualize this part radiating light and strength, spreading throughout your entire body. Let this energy fill you, symbolizing your feminine essence and resilience.

Redefining Your Own Story

Ultimately, this journey is about reclaiming the story of who you are and embracing a femininity that is uniquely yours. You are not defined by what society believes femininity should be; you are defined by what you believe it is. Allow yourself to own this narrative, to live by your own standards, and to let go of any limitations that once held you back.

As you redefine femininity on your terms, remember that your story is beautiful and complete as it is. You are a woman with depth, creativity, wisdom, and strength a woman who has chosen to live as her true self, unapologetically and fully. This chapter is a celebration of your journey, a reminder that femininity is yours to define, yours to embody, and yours to own in every way that feels right to you.

6

Chapter 6: Channeling Instead of Escaping

When life feels overwhelming, it's natural to want to escape, to turn away from the intensity of our emotions and seek relief in anything that helps us feel "outside" of ourselves. But there's a power far greater than escape and that's channeling. When we channel, we direct our emotions, pain, and energy into something meaningful, transforming difficult feelings into tools for growth and healing. Rather than running from ourselves, we learn to hold space for everything we feel, allowing it to become a source of insight and strength.

In this chapter, we'll explore alternative mental health practices that help us channel rather than escape. This isn't about pushing away our feelings or bypassing our pain; it's about finding ways to express, process, and understand ourselves on a deeper level. When we channel our energy, we turn it into a force that grounds us, centers us, and ultimately brings us closer to peace.

Creative Outlets as Healing Tools

Art, music, and writing are powerful ways to channel our emotions into something tangible. When words feel insufficient, painting or drawing can help us express feelings that are otherwise hard to define. The act of creating whether it's with a brush, an instrument, or a pen gives our emotions a voice and a form. We don't have to be artists or musicians to find healing in these practices; we only need to show up, allowing ourselves to create without judgment or expectation.

- **Art**: Whether it's painting, sketching, or even collaging, visual art can help us externalize our inner world. As you create, let go of any need for perfection or "skill" he goal is simply to give shape to what you feel.

- **Music**: Listening to music can soothe the spirit, but making music whether through singing, playing an instrument, or even humming along creates a deep connection between body and soul. Music has a way of holding space for our feelings, allowing us to express what words often can't.

- **Writing**: Journaling or free-writing is an incredibly grounding practice. By putting our thoughts onto paper, we give them a place to rest outside of our minds. Write without censoring yourself, letting your thoughts and emotions flow freely.

These creative outlets remind us that we have the power to transform our pain into beauty, our confusion into clarity. Channeling through art, music, and writing allows us to connect to ourselves in a way that's honest and unfiltered, giving us a safe space to explore our emotions.

Grounding Practices for Reconnecting with Your Body

Channeling is not just about expressing emotions; it's also about staying connected to our bodies, anchoring ourselves in the present moment. Grounding practices help us find stability, especially when life feels chaotic. They remind us that, no matter what's happening around us, we have the power to create a sense of calm within.

- **Breathwork**: Conscious breathing is one of the simplest and most effective grounding tools. Try inhaling deeply, holding the breath for a few moments, and then exhaling slowly. Focus on each breath, allowing it to bring you back into your body.

- **Body Scanning**: Take a few moments to mentally "scan" your body from head to toe, noticing any areas of tension or discomfort. Imagine releasing that tension with each exhale, letting your body feel relaxed and supported.

- **Nature Connection**: Spending time outdoors, even if it's just a short walk or sitting in the sun, helps ground us. Nature has a way of calming the mind and reconnecting us to a sense of peace. Touching the earth, feeling the wind, or listening to the sounds around you can be deeply grounding.

- **Physical Movement**: Gentle movement, like stretching or yoga, allows us to reconnect with our bodies. Focus on each movement, noticing how it feels and releasing any tension as you go.

These grounding practices remind us that we are more than our thoughts and emotions; we are whole beings capable of creating calm within ourselves.

Meditation and Mindfulness for Inner Peace

Mindfulness and meditation teach us to observe our thoughts and feelings without getting lost in them. These practices create a sense of inner stillness, helping us reconnect with ourselves and find peace, regardless of what's happening around us.

- **Meditation**: Start with just a few minutes each day, sitting quietly and focusing on your breath. Notice any thoughts or feelings that come up, but try not to engage with them. Simply observe, allowing each thought to pass like a cloud in the sky.

- **Mindful Moments**: Incorporate mindfulness into your daily routine by bringing your full attention to simple activities, like washing your hands, drinking a cup of tea, or walking. Notice each sensation, sound, and feeling, allowing yourself to be fully present.

- **Gratitude Practice**: Taking a few moments each day to reflect on what you're grateful for can shift your perspective, helping you focus on the positive aspects of your life.

Mindfulness and meditation don't make our challenges disappear, but they give us the ability to remain calm and centered, even in difficult moments. By observing our thoughts and emotions without attachment, we create space between ourselves and our struggles, allowing us to respond with clarity and compassion.

Choosing Inner Peace as a Daily Ritual

Ultimately, channeling instead of escaping is about choosing inner peace as a way of life. This peace isn't conditional it's not dependent on what's happening outside of us. Instead, it's a choice we make every day, a commitment to cultivate calm, clarity, and acceptance within ourselves.

- **Create a Daily Ritual**: Set aside time each day to connect with yourself, whether it's through journaling, meditation, or simply sitting quietly. Let this time be a sacred space where you can let go of the day's stresses and return to a state of peace.

· **Practice Self-Compassion**: When you feel overwhelmed, speak to yourself with kindness. Remind yourself that you are doing your best and that it's okay to feel what you're feeling.

· **Reflect on Your Journey**: Take moments to acknowledge how far you've come, the challenges you've faced, and the growth you've experienced. Recognize that your journey is unique and that you have the power to create peace within it.

Inner peace is not something we find; it's something we create. When we choose to channel rather than escape, we honor our experiences and allow them to become part of our healing. By grounding ourselves, expressing our emotions, and cultivating mindfulness, we build a foundation of resilience and calm that can carry us through anything life brings.

This chapter is a guide to discovering the power of channeling, the beauty of grounding, and the strength of inner peace. With each practice, we reclaim our power, not by escaping from ourselves, but by choosing to be fully present, fully alive, and fully at peace

7

Chapter 7: The Power of Self-Acceptance and Ownership

Self-acceptance is one of the most liberating gifts we can give ourselves. It's about looking at who we are, in every phase of life, and saying, *"This is me, and I embrace every part of my journey."* Radical self-acceptance means we stop waiting to be "better," thinner, more accomplished, or somehow more worthy. We choose, instead, to see ourselves with compassion, to honor the unique paths we're on, and to own every part of who we are flaws, strengths, and all.

The power of self-acceptance lies in its ability to make us whole. When we accept ourselves fully, we no longer feel fragmented, as though parts of us need to be hidden or changed to be worthy of love. We recognize that we are enough just as we are. This chapter is a journey into what it means to live with self-acceptance and ownership, exploring how self-compassion, authenticity, and honesty create a foundation for true empowerment.

Embracing Radical Self-Acceptance

Radical self-acceptance isn't just about acknowledging the parts of ourselves we like—it's about embracing all of who we are, including the aspects we might struggle with. It's understanding that we don't have to be "perfect" to be worthy, that our value doesn't come from meeting society's standards but from our own recognition of our worth. This kind of acceptance allows us to step into our power, to walk through life with confidence, and to face challenges knowing that, no matter what, we are enough.

To live with self-acceptance is to give ourselves permission to grow and change at our own pace. It's understanding that we're allowed to be works in progress, that we can love ourselves today, even as we work toward becoming who we want to be tomorrow. This acceptance creates an inner peace, a quiet strength that can't be shaken by the opinions of others or by life's inevitable ups and downs.

Self-Compassion, Authenticity, and Honesty as Empowerment Tools

Self-compassion is the practice of treating ourselves with the same kindness we would extend to a dear friend. Instead of criticizing ourselves for every perceived flaw or mistake, we learn to offer understanding, to acknowledge that we are human, and to release the harsh judgments that only weigh us down. Self-compassion allows us to move through life with a softer, more forgiving heart, creating a safe space within ourselves where we can grow without fear of condemnation.

Authenticity is about being real, about showing up in life as our true selves rather than hiding behind masks or pretending to be something we're not. When we are authentic, we align with our inner truth, speaking, acting, and living in ways that are genuine. Authenticity empowers us because it frees us from the exhausting task of maintaining a facade, allowing us to use our energy for what truly matters—living a life that feels meaningful and true.

Honesty with ourselves is a powerful tool for growth. It means being willing to see and accept our own patterns, strengths, and areas for growth. By being honest with ourselves, we stop running from the parts of our lives that are difficult or uncomfortable, and we take ownership of our choices. Honesty grounds us in reality and empowers us to make conscious, intentional decisions about who we want to become.

Embracing the Journey: Strength in Healing, Rebuilding, and Thriving

The journey of self-acceptance is not a straight line. It's a path that includes moments of doubt, setbacks, and growth. But within each phase of this journey lies the strength to heal, rebuild, and ultimately thrive. True self-acceptance is not a destination; it's a practice we return to every day. There will be days when we feel empowered, confident, and fully at ease with ourselves, and other days when we struggle. But in both moments, we have the opportunity to choose acceptance, to trust that every phase of our lives is necessary and valuable.

Healing is an act of courage. It takes strength to face our pain, to confront the wounds we carry, and to give ourselves permission to move forward. Rebuilding is an act of faith. It requires us to let go of who we thought we needed to be, creating space for who we are becoming. And thriving is an act of self-love. It's the result of embracing the fullness of our lives, of knowing that we are worthy of joy, peace, and fulfillment.

Each step on this journey builds our strength, shaping us into resilient, empowered individuals who own their lives with confidence. By accepting ourselves fully, we create a foundation that allows us to thrive, no matter what life brings our way.

Reflections and Affirmations for Self-Acceptance and Ownership

As you continue this journey, it can be helpful to pause and reflect, to remind yourself of the progress you've made and the commitment you hold to honor yourself. Here are some reflections and affirmations to guide you in owning your path, your body, and your power.

I am worthy of love and acceptance in every phase of my life.

- Remind yourself that worthiness is not something you earn; it's something that is inherent to you, simply because you exist.

I choose to embrace myself fully, flaws and all.

- Remember that each part of you, even the parts you may struggle with, is worthy of acceptance and compassion.

I honor my journey and trust in the growth it brings.

- Acknowledge that your life's journey is unique, with its own rhythm and timing, and that each step is a part of your growth.

I am committed to living authentically and honoring my truth.

- Remind yourself that your truth matters, and that living authentically is a powerful act of self-respect.

I release the need for perfection and embrace myself as I am.

- Allow yourself to let go of the pressure to be "perfect" and recognize that you are enough just as you are.

I am resilient, capable, and whole.

- Affirm that you have the strength to face whatever comes, that you are complete, and that you are capable of creating a life of fulfillment.

-

Owning Your Path, Body, and Power

This chapter is an invitation to live with self-acceptance and ownership, to choose radical compassion for yourself, and to trust in the power that comes from honoring your journey.

Embrace who you are in every phase of life, knowing that your path, your body, and your power are sacred. When you choose to accept yourself fully, you not only free yourself from the weight of others' expectations, but you also step into a life of true empowerment.

Self-acceptance and ownership are not just acts of self-love; they are the foundation of resilience, the keys to a life lived in peace and authenticity. Through this journey, may you come to see yourself with eyes of love and respect, owning every part of your story and celebrating the strength, beauty, and power that is uniquely yours.

8

Chapter 8: Living as Dangerous Pussi

Living as "Dangerous Pussi" means embracing life with unapologetic boldness, a fierce love for yourself, and an unwavering commitment to owning every part of who you are. It's about standing tall, rooted in the knowledge that your power lies in your authenticity and your courage to live beyond the limitations others might place upon you. Living this way isn't about defying society just for the sake of rebellion it's about allowing yourself to exist fully and fiercely, without fear or apology.

To live as Dangerous Pussi is to embrace the fire within, the part of you that longs to live out loud, to express yourself freely, and to honor every facet of your being. It's the embodiment of self-love, self-respect, and self-confidence, a life lived with purpose and joy. In this chapter, we'll explore what it means to live boldly, let go of societal expectations, and fully celebrate the beauty of your body, mind, and spirit.

Embracing All Facets of Yourself with Unapologetic Boldness

Boldness is not about being fearless; it's about moving forward even when fear tries to hold you back. Living boldly means giving yourself permission to be fully seen, to speak your truth, and to trust in your worthiness, even if it makes others uncomfortable. It's about choosing to be your truest self, even if that self doesn't fit neatly into society's expectations.

Being unapologetically bold requires you to stop seeking external validation. You are no longer waiting for permission to be yourself, to take up space, or to go after what you desire. You are giving yourself permission to be exactly who you are, knowing that your power comes from your authenticity. When you live this way, you inspire others to do the same. Your boldness becomes a light, a reminder that there is nothing more beautiful than a person who is fully, unapologetically themselves.

Tips for Connecting to Your Inner Fire and Letting Go of Societal Expectations

Living as Dangerous Pussi means connecting to the fire within-inthe deep, passionate energy that drives you, fuels you, and gives you a sense of purpose. This inner fire is your vitality, your enthusiasm, and your desire to live life on your terms. To connect with it, you must be willing to let go of the limiting beliefs and expectations society has placed upon you.

Identify What Sets Your Soul on Fire: What makes you feel alive? What are the activities, people, or passions that bring you the most joy and fulfillment? Make a list, and commit to incorporating these things into your life as much as possible.

Release External Approval: Recognize where you're holding onto the need for others' approval. Practice letting go of this need by making decisions based on what feels right for you, rather than what you think others will accept or praise.

Set Boundaries with Confidence: Living boldly requires boundaries. Be clear about what you will and won't accept in your life, and hold firm to these boundaries. This allows you to protect your energy and focus on the things that truly matter to you.

Challenge Limiting Beliefs: Identify beliefs that are holding you back from being fully yourself. Ask yourself, *Is this belief truly mine, or has it been imposed by society, family, or culture?* Replace these limiting beliefs with empowering truths that align with who you want to be.

Celebrate Your Uniqueness: Embrace the parts of yourself that make you different. Celebrate the quirks, preferences, and passions that make you who you are. Let go of any pressure to conform, knowing that your individuality is your strength.

*Celebrating the Body, Mind, and Spirit as a Whole and
Powerful Entity*

Living as Dangerous Pussi means celebrating yourself as a
complete being. Your body, mind, and spirit are not separate
they are interconnected parts of the powerful whole that is *you*.
By honoring and nurturing each of these aspects, you create a
foundation of strength, resilience, and inner peace.

- **Celebrate Your Body**: Your body is your sacred vessel, de-
  serving of love, care, and appreciation. Instead of focusing
  on societal ideals of beauty, focus on how your body feels,
  how it supports you, and the experiences it allows you to
  have. Take time each day to express gratitude for your body,
  treating it with kindness and respect.

- **Nourish Your Mind**: Feed your mind with thoughts, ideas,
  and knowledge that uplift and empower you. Challenge
  yourself to explore new perspectives, learn new things, and
  keep an open mind. Protect your mental well-being by
  setting boundaries around the information and energies
  you allow into your life.

- **Honor Your Spirit**: Your spirit is the essence of who you
  are the part of you that is connected to something greater,
  whether that be nature, the universe, or the divine. Find

ways to nurture this connection through practices that resonate with you, such as meditation, prayer, nature walks, or creative expression. Embracing your spiritual essence helps you tap into a sense of purpose and inner peace.

When you see yourself as a whole being body, mind, and spirit you begin to understand your true power. You are not just a collection of parts; you are a dynamic, interconnected being capable of extraordinary things.

Leading with Confidence, Wisdom, and Fierce Love

Living as Dangerous Pussi is an act of leadership. It's about showing up in life with confidence, using your wisdom to guide you, and leading with fierce love for yourself and others. Confidence comes from knowing who you are and owning it fully. Wisdom comes from honoring your experiences and trusting the lessons you've learned. And fierce love is the fuel that sustains you, reminding you that, above all else, you deserve to live a life that feels true and fulfilling.

Lead with Confidence: Trust in your worth, your voice, and your abilities. When you lead with confidence, you inspire others to believe in themselves as well. Remember that confidence is not about perfection it's about showing up as you are and trusting that you are enough.

Embrace Your Wisdom: Every experience you've had has

brought you wisdom. Embrace the lessons life has taught you, and use them to navigate future challenges with grace. Your wisdom is your gift, your guide, and your anchor.

Love Fiercely: Love yourself fiercely, without conditions. Love others fiercely, allowing them the freedom to be themselves. And love life fiercely, embracing its beauty and its challenges with an open heart.

Living as Dangerous Pussi is about reclaiming the fullness of who you are. It's about stepping into your power, celebrating your uniqueness, and leading a life that feels aligned, purposeful, and free. This chapter is an invitation to live boldly, to let go of limitations, and to trust that you are powerful beyond measure.

As you move forward, let each day be a celebration of the woman you are becoming. Stand tall in your truth, embrace your inner fire, and know that you have everything within you to live a life of confidence, wisdom, and fierce love. Because that's what it means to be Dangerous Pussi a woman who lives fearlessly, loves deeply, and owns her power in every sense of the word.

9

Special Bonus Special Chapter 9: Dangerous Steps to Healing Sexual Trauma and Abuse

Healing from sexual trauma isn't linear, pretty, or easy but damn, it's powerful. These five steps are not about "fixing" yourself, because you're not broken. They're about reclaiming, rebuilding, and rising into the dangerous, unapologetic force you were always meant to be. Let's get to it.

Step 1: Face the Shadow

"You can't heal what you won't feel."

Listen, you can't keep running from the pain and expect to find peace. That darkness you're avoiding? It's waiting for you to look it in the eye. It's not here to break you; it's here to teach you. Healing starts when you stop numbing and start feeling.

Take a deep breath and dive in. The hurt, the anger, the shame it's messy, and it's heavy, but it's real. And real is where the magic happens. You've got to sit with it, even when it feels unbearable, because ignoring it only gives it more power over you.

How to Do It:

- Grab a journal, a pen, and a quiet space.
- Write the unfiltered truth. Not the sugar-coated version, but the raw, jagged-edged stuff that makes your heart race just thinking about it.
- Ask yourself:
- When did I first feel powerless?
- What am I afraid to admit, even to myself?
- What do I need to release to reclaim my strength?

Don't hold back. Cry, scream, rip the pages if you need to. Let it all out, because that's the first step to breaking free.

Mantra for the Shadow Work:
"I will no longer fear my pain. It is a part of me, but it does not define me."
Facing the shadow is like walking through fire, but on the other side? Baby, that's where the healing begins. This is your moment to be brave.

Step 2: Break the Silence

"Your voice is your first weapon of defense, and it's time to sharpen it."

Let me tell you something: silence is a prison, and shame is the warden. The longer you keep your story locked up, the more it eats away at you. But here's the truth they don't win when you speak. The moment you let your voice out, that shame starts crumbling.

Speak your truth. Whisper it, shout it, write it down, or cry it into the wind. It doesn't have to be pretty or perfect it just has to be *yours.* Find someone you trust, even if that someone is just the reflection staring back at you. Look her in the eye and say, *"I've been hurt, but I'm still here."*

How to Do It:

- Start small: Write a letter to yourself or someone who hurt you. You don't have to send it this is for you.
- Record yourself: talking about what happened. Play it back and remind yourself: *This is my story, and I own it.*
- Share with someone safe :a therapist, a trusted friend, or even your journal. Breaking the silence doesn't mean shouting from the rooftops (unless you want to). It's about releasing that energy and letting it breathe.

Why It Matters:

When you speak your truth, you claim it. It stops being something that happened *to* you and starts being something you survived. Your voice is more powerful than you know it's the tool that sets you free.

Mantra for Breaking the Silence:

"I am not my secrets. I am my strength. My voice is my freedom."

Let the words out, no matter how shaky or small they feel. Trust me, they'll grow stronger, and so will you. You're not just breaking silence you're breaking chains.

Step 4: Build Sacred Boundaries

"Protect your peace like your life depends on it...because it does."

Let me make one thing crystal clear: boundaries are not rude, selfish, or mean. Boundaries are *sacred*. They're the armor you wear to protect your energy, your heart, and your sanity. Without them, you're letting anyone and everyone walk through your door with muddy boots and bad intentions. Nope. Not anymore.

It's time to draw the line. Not a pencil line they can erase, but a bold, unbreakable boundary that says, *"This is my space, my time, my energy—and I decide who gets access."*

How to Do It:
Define Your Non-Negotiables

- Ask yourself: *What drains me? What lifts me up?* Write down what you absolutely will not tolerate in relationships, work, and even with yourself.

Say No Without Guilt

- Practice saying "no" in front of the mirror if you have to. No explanations, no apologies. Just *"No, that doesn't work for me."*

Create Energy Checkpoints

- At the end of each day, ask yourself: *Did I honor my boundaries today? Did I protect my peace?* If not, adjust tomorrow.

Communicate Clearly

- Don't expect people to read your mind. Tell them what's okay and what's not. And if they don't respect it? Bye.

Honor Your Own Rules

- The hardest part is keeping boundaries with yourself. If you say you're taking a break, take it. If you say you're done with toxic people, be done. Show yourself the same respect you demand from others.

Why It Matters:

Boundaries aren't just about keeping the bad out; they're about making room for the good. When you set limits, you protect your energy for the things that truly matter—your healing, your growth, and your joy.

Mantra for Boundaries:

"My energy is sacred. My peace is non-negotiable. I am worthy

of respect and protection."

Trust me, once you start enforcing boundaries, you'll see the world and yourself differently. You'll stop apologizing for taking up space and start demanding the treatment you deserve. And honey, that's dangerous in the best possible way.

Step 5: Redefine Pleasure and Power

"Your fire didn't die, it just needs oxygen to roar again."

Let's talk about pleasure, not just the kind that makes you blush, but the kind that makes you feel *alive.* After trauma, pleasure can feel like a foreign language, something out of reach or even scary. But here's the truth: pleasure is your birthright. It's not just about feeling good, it's about reclaiming the joy, power, and connection that were always yours.

Redefining pleasure means creating it for yourself, on your terms. It's not about anyone else's expectations, desires, or opinions. It's about what makes *you* feel powerful, beautiful, and whole again.

How to Do It:
Start with Curiosity

- Ask yourself: *What lights me up? What makes me smile? What feels good to my body and soul?* Explore without judgment or pressure.

Explore Sensuality Without Shame

- Light candles, wear fabrics that feel divine, play music that moves you. Sensuality isn't just physical—it's in the way you connect with the world around you.

Celebrate Small Pleasures

- Savor the taste of your favorite food. Feel the sun on your skin. Dance in your kitchen. These small moments of joy are where healing begins.

Reclaim Your Power Through Pleasure

- Understand that your joy and pleasure are revolutionary acts. They're proof that trauma didn't win, that you're still standing, still thriving, still *you.*

Give Yourself Permission

- Permission to feel. Permission to want. Permission to be messy, loud, and unapologetically you. Stop waiting for someone else to validate your happiness it's already yours.

Why It Matters:

Pleasure isn't just about indulgence it's about survival. It's about reminding yourself that life can be beautiful again, that your body can feel like home, and that your spirit can burn bright. Pleasure is power, and it's time to own both.

Mantra for Redefining Pleasure:

"I deserve joy. I deserve pleasure. I deserve to live fully, fiercely, and unapologetically."

This is your moment to take back everything trauma tried to steal. You're not just surviving you're thriving. You're dangerous, divine, and unstoppable. Let the world feel your fire.

Special Mention: Existential Kink

Let me put you on to something: *Existential Kink* by Carolyn Elliott is not your typical self-help book. It's a permission slip to dive into the shadows and *love* what you find there. This book flips the script on healing by teaching you how to embrace the parts of yourself you've been told to hidethe messy, the taboo, the parts you think are too "broken" to fix.

Elliott's approach is bold, raw, and yes, kinky but not in the way you might think. It's about finding the pleasure in the pain, the beauty in the chaos, and the power in your darkest desires. This isn't just about healing; it's about transforming the way you see yourself and your life.

Why It's a Game-Changer

- It's not afraid to go where most books won't: into the depths of your subconscious, where your shame, fear, and guilt live.

- It shows you how to reclaim your shadow—those hidden,

"forbidden" parts of yourself—and turn them into sources of strength and joy.

- It's a wild, unapologetic ride that challenges you to own every piece of who you are, even the ones you'd rather leave behind.

The Therapy of It All

Here's the thing: *Existential Kink* isn't just a book; it's a practice. The exercises in it guide you to literally *feel good* about the stuff you hate. Sound crazy? It kind of is but in the best way. It's about flipping the switch and realizing that even your pain is a part of your power.

This book pairs perfectly with the themes in *Dangerous Pussi* because it reminds you that healing isn't about running from the darkness it's about dancing in it. It's about finding pleasure in places you never thought possible and owning your story with bold, unapologetic pride.

If you're ready to see your trauma, desires, and life in a whole new way, give *Existential Kink* a read. Trust me, it's dangerous in the best way possible.

10

Conclusion

Conclusion: The Rebirth of Self and Spirit

As we reach the end of this journey, we find ourselves standing in the light of a profound rebirth a rebirth of self and spirit that comes from embracing our true power, even in the face of profound change. For those of us who have experienced a hysterectomy, the path to reclaiming feminine power is unique, often filled with deep reflection, vulnerability, and healing. But this journey is also a testament to our resilience, a testament to the unbreakable spirit within each of us.

Owning our power after a hysterectomy is about more than simply accepting what's changed; it's about redefining our own vision of femininity and strength. It's about letting go of the limitations that once held us back and celebrating every part of who we are. Through this journey, we have embraced the art of surrender, chosen to channel rather than escape, and learned to honor our bodies, minds, and spirits as powerful, interconnected entities.

This rebirth is a reminder that transformation is a part of life's natural rhythm. There is beauty in change, strength in growth, and freedom in acceptance. We have come to understand that our true power doesn't lie in meeting others' expectations but in fully accepting and loving ourselves as we are. This journey has shown us that femininity is not defined by any single part of us; it is an energy, a force, a spirit that radiates from the core of who we are.

As you continue forward, know that you carry within you all the wisdom, strength, and love you need to walk confidently in your truth. The experiences you've had, the challenges you've faced, and the growth you've achieved have shaped you into a woman who is not only powerful but also deeply connected to her own soul. You are living proof of the beauty that arises from transformation, the light that shines through even the darkest moments.

May you continue to walk in your truth, grounded in the knowledge of your worth and the strength of your journey. Embrace the freedom that comes from living as your fullest, most authentic self. Celebrate the rebirth of your spirit, and let it be a guide as you move forward, filled with purpose, passion, and fierce love for yourself and for life.

This rebirth is not an ending; it is a new beginning. May it inspire you to live boldly, to love deeply, and to embrace each moment as a celebration of the powerful, beautiful, and resilient woman you are. Because in the end, that is what it means to truly live free, fearless, and fully alive.

Epilogue

Preparation and Care for a Vaginal Total Hysterectomy and Abdominal Hysterectomy

When facing a procedure as significant as a vaginal total hysterectomy or an abdominal hysterectomy, it's important to feel prepared, informed, and empowered at every stage. I believe that knowledge is power, and caring for yourself through this journey is both a physical and spiritual process. I'll walk you through the preparation, the middle (surgery day), and the after-care so that you can move forward with confidence and compassion for yourself.

Before: Preparing Your Mind, Body, and Spirit

Educate Yourself, but Don't Overwhelm Yourself

- Read up on what the procedures involve, but try to stick to reputable sources. A little knowledge can ease anxiety, but too much digging can sometimes lead to unnecessary worry.

- Understand the purpose and potential outcomes. For a

vaginal total hysterectomy, you're looking at the removal of your uterus and cervix, sometimes along with the Fallopian tubes and ovaries. An abdominal hysterectomy typically involves an exploratory or corrective look into the uterus through a small incision, often with minimal removal of tissue.

Emotional Preparation

- Take a moment to honor the journey you're on. Many women feel a range of emotions leading up to these surgeries grief, relief, anxiety, and hope. These are all natural. Give yourself permission to feel them without judgment.

- Write down any fears or hopes you have. This is a time to get clear on what you need emotionally, spiritually, and mentally. Setting intentions before the procedure can help you feel grounded and in control.

Physical Preparation

- **Health and Nutrition**: Leading up to surgery, nourish your body with balanced meals rich in vitamins, protein, and minerals to support healing. Hydration is equally important; it can help with post-surgery recovery and prevent complications.

- **Pre-Surgery Checklist**: Your doctor may ask you to avoid certain medications, alcohol, or heavy foods in the days prior. Follow these guidelines carefully. You might also be instructed to fast the night before.

- **Prepare Your Home**: Stock up on comfortable foods, easy-to-wear clothing, and any hygiene or medical items (pads, abdominal pillows, loose underwear) that will aid in your recovery. Consider arranging things within arm's reach to avoid unnecessary stretching or bending.

Support System

- Let your close ones know what you're going through. Enlist someone who can drive you to and from the hospital, and maybe have a friend or family member stay with you for the first few days after you're home.
- Make sure to prepare your support system for the different levels of care you'll need physically and emotionally.
-

Middle: Surgery Day

Mental Grounding

- This is a big day, and it's normal to feel a mix of emotions. Begin with a few deep breaths to center yourself. Remind yourself why you're doing this, and focus on the healing to come.

- Affirmations or prayer can be helpful to ground yourself. Something as simple as, "I am safe. I am healing. I am in good hands," can bring calm before going under anesthesia.

Arrival and Pre-Surgery Routine

- Upon arrival, you'll be checked in and asked to change into surgical attire. You'll have per-operative checks, including blood pressure, temperature, and any final questions with your doctor or anesthesiologist.

- Remember to advocate for yourself here if you have any last-minute concerns or clarifications. The medical team is there to support you, so make sure you're clear about any allergies, anxieties, or special requests.

- As you're prepped for surgery, try to focus on your breath and remind yourself that this is a step toward healing and renewal.

Surgery

- For a vaginal total hysterectomy, the surgeon will remove the uterus through the vagina, possibly along with the cervix, Fallopian tubes, and ovaries if specified. For an abdominal hysterectomy, a small incision is made, usually around the navel, to allow the surgeon to examine and possibly treat areas within the uterus.

- While you're under anesthesia, your body is in the hands of a skilled team working with precision and care. Trust in the process and the professionals around you.

After: Healing and Recovery

Immediate Post-Surgery

- In the recovery room, you'll gradually come out of anesthesia. You may feel groggy, disoriented, or even emotional. These are normal responses and usually subside as your body metabolizes the anesthesia.

- Pain and nausea are common right after surgery. The nurses will monitor you closely, and they'll provide pain management as needed. Communicate with them about your pain levels this is not the time to "tough it out."

- Expect to stay a few hours to a day depending on the complexity of your procedure and how you're recovering.

At-Home Recovery
Physical Care

- **Rest and Gentle Movement**: Rest is essential, but gentle movement—like short, slow walks around your home helps prevent stiffness and improves circulation. Listen to your body, and don't push it too far too soon.

- **Managing Pain**: Take prescribed medications as directed. Don't hesitate to use heat pads (if recommended by your doctor) or abdominal pillows to reduce pain or pressure.

- **Hygiene and Wound Care**: Keep any incision sites clean and dry. For the first few weeks, avoid heavy lifting, strenuous activities, and anything that could strain your abdominal or pelvic area. Your doctor will give you specific guidelines, so follow these closely.

- **Diet**: Eat light, nourishing meals. Fiber-rich foods, fluids, and gentle herbal teas like chamomile or ginger can aid in digestion and reduce discomfort.

Emotional and Spiritual Care

- **Honor Your Feelings**: You may feel a range of emotions post-surgery, from relief to grief. Acknowledge these without judgment, and give yourself space to process them. Journaling, meditating, or simply talking with a supportive friend can help.

- **Connecting with Your Body**: Practice gentle self-compassion exercises like affirmations or meditative breathing, sending gratitude to your body for its resilience and strength. Reclaiming your body as a whole, beautiful, and powerful vessel can be a healing ritual as you adapt to this new chapter.

Reconnect with Your Feminine Energy

- Just because parts of your body have changed doesn't mean your femininity has. Find small ways to honor your feminine spirit through art, nature, rituals, or whatever else brings you joy and a sense of self. This is an empowering time to rediscover what makes you feel connected to yourself.

Follow-Up and Long-Term Healing

- Regular follow-ups are key. Your doctor will assess your healing and discuss any long-term care. If you experience unusual symptoms like severe pain, fever, or abnormal bleeding contact your medical team immediately.

- Your energy levels may take time to return, and hormonal changes can influence your mood, skin, and more. Be patient with yourself, and don't be afraid to ask for additional support if you need it, whether it's hormonal support, physical therapy, or emotional counseling.

Embracing Your New Chapter

A vaginal total hysterectomy or abdominal hysterectomy is a powerful journey of healing, one that invites you to redefine your relationship with your body and spirit. This process is about more than physical recovery; it's about honoring yourself, accepting your resilience, and embracing this new chapter with strength and self-love.

Afterword

Understanding Complications and Practical Recovery Tips

As with any surgery, a vaginal total hysterectomy or abdominal hysterectomy can come with its own set of potential complications, but being aware and prepared can make all the difference. Here's a look at some possible complications to keep on your radar, as well as practical steps to aid in your recovery. Think of this as your guide to both staying safe and supporting your healing in real, doable ways.

Potential Complications to Watch Out For

Infection:

- This is one of the most common post-surgery concerns. Watch for signs like redness, warmth, or swelling around any incision sites, as well as a fever or unusual discharge. These can signal an infection and require immediate attention.

- **Practical Tip**: Keep your incision sites clean and dry. Follow your doctor's instructions on how to care for these areas, and avoid soaking in baths or swimming until you're cleared to do so.

Heavy Bleeding:

- Light bleeding or spotting is normal after a hysterectomy, but anything that looks like a heavy period (or worse) should be reported. Heavy bleeding could indicate complications with the healing process, and it's important not to ignore it.

- **Practical Tip**: Use only pads no tampons to monitor bleeding. Avoid activities that might put strain on the pelvic area, such as lifting heavy objects or overexerting yourself too soon.

Blood Clots:

- Surgery can increase the risk of blood clots, especially in the legs. Swelling, redness, or tenderness in your calves, as well as shortness of breath, should be taken seriously as they might indicate a clot.

- **Practical Tip**: Gentle movement is your friend. Short walks around the house and leg exercises (like simple ankle circles or gentle stretches) can help maintain circulation. Aim to get up and move a bit every few hours, even if it's just to stand and stretch.

Pain and Discomfort:

- While some pain is to be expected, sharp or worsening pain that doesn't respond to prescribed medications could indicate an issue, like internal bleeding or nerve complications.

- **Practical Tip**: Stay on top of your pain meds as prescribed, especially in the first few days when you'll need them most. Heat packs (if approved) or abdominal pillows can provide additional comfort.

-

Constipation:

- After anesthesia and pain medications, constipation can be a frustrating but common issue. Straining too much can interfere with healing, so it's best to handle this proactively.

- **Practical Tip**: Add fiber-rich foods to your diet, drink plenty of water, and don't shy away from a gentle stool softener if your doctor approves. Warm herbal teas, especially those with ginger or peppermint, can also soothe digestion.

Urinary Issues:

- Some women experience difficulty urinating after surgery, either due to temporary nerve impacts or because the area around the bladder may be sensitive.

- **Practical Tip**: Try to stay calm if you find urination a bit challenging. Sometimes, sitting forward slightly or running warm water in the sink can help relax the bladder. Keep an eye out for any burning or painful urination, as this could indicate a urinary tract infection.

Practical Tips to Aid Recovery

Rest and Honor Your Pace:

- Your body has just undergone a major experience, and it needs time to heal. Avoid any temptation to push yourself to "get back to normal" quickly.

- **Practical Tip**: Make your recovery time a sacred space. Set up a comfortable area with everything you need within reach water, your phone, books, snacks, and medications. Embrace this time to rest without guilt.

Listen to Your Body's Limits:

- It's easy to forget that even if you *feel* okay, your body is still healing. Avoid heavy lifting, bending, or standing for long periods for the first few weeks.

- **Practical Tip**: Accept help from others and don't feel guilty for saying "no" to anything physically demanding. If something doesn't feel right or causes discomfort, listen to that signal and back off.

Nourish Yourself with Healing Foods:

- Fuel your body with foods that support recovery. High-protein foods help repair tissues, and antioxidant-rich fruits and vegetables support your immune system.

- **Practical Tip**: Think of meals as a form of medicine. Soups, smoothies, and easy-to-digest meals with plenty of lean protein (like chicken, fish, or legumes) will help you feel good and keep your energy up.

Stay Hydrated:

- Hydration is essential, especially if you're dealing with any post-op medications or discomfort. Water helps flush out toxins, supports your immune system, and prevents constipation.

- **Practical Tip**: Keep a large water bottle nearby and sip on it throughout the day. Herbal teas or water with a splash of lemon or cucumber can make it easier to get enough fluids.

Practice Gentle Movement:

- When you're ready, light movement can do wonders for your circulation and mental health. Short, gentle walks around your home or yard can help prevent stiffness and improve mood.

- **Practical Tip**: Set small movement goals, like a two-minute walk every few hours, then gradually increase as you feel able. Just moving your body in small ways can ease tension and improve blood flow.

Mental and Emotional Care:

- Surgery can impact your emotions, and it's perfectly normal to feel everything from relief to sadness. Allow yourself the full range of emotions.

- **Practical Tip**: Journaling, meditation, or talking with loved ones can help you process any emotional waves. Consider reaching out to a support group or therapist if you feel that would benefit your healing.

Set Up Follow-Up Appointments:

- Recovery is ongoing, and follow-ups help ensure you're healing properly. Be proactive about scheduling these appointments and be open with your doctor about any lingering symptoms or questions.

- **Practical Tip**: Before each visit, jot down any symptoms or concerns you want to discuss. Don't feel pressured to "tough it out" your doctor is there to help ensure your comfort and well-being.

This is a journey, and your body deserves care, patience, and gentleness as you heal. By staying mindful of these potential complications and honoring your body's needs with practical steps, you're giving yourself the best chance at a smooth and empowered recovery. And remember, this is *your* time to heal both physically and emotionally so embrace each day with grace and compassion for yourself. You're doing beautifully.

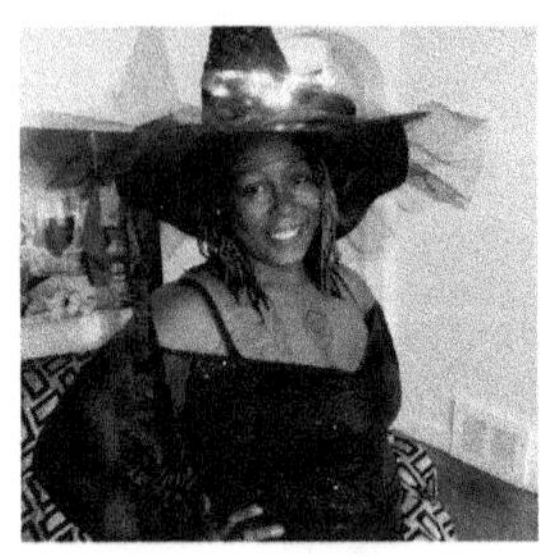

About the Author

Icy Kendrick is a visionary psychic medium, spiritual guide, and creator of *Divine Pause Oasis*, a sanctuary for self-discovery and spiritual transformation. Born and raised in Detroit, Michigan, Icy combines her deep-rooted spiritual gifts with the strength and resilience she cultivated in her vibrant hometown. With an intuitive mastery of Numerology, Tarot, Astrology, and the profound wisdom of the Bible, Icy offers a unique fusion of modern spirituality and ancient insight, guiding clients toward emotional healing, clarity, and a deeper connection with Spirit.

Icy brings a compassionate, grounded perspective to her work, offering 1-on-1 private readings and enriching group sessions designed especially for professional women and stay-at-home mothers seeking to rediscover their true essence and awaken their spiritual potential. Her approach invites clients to pause, reflect, and journey into self-discovery with openness and wonder. Known for her profound insights and heart-centered guidance, Icy empowers clients to embrace their authentic selves, fostering resilience, confidence, and alignment with their higher purpose.

Through *Divine Pause Oasis*, Icy has created a community where women are inspired to live with passion, purpose, and clarity. She also offers access to transformative programs like *Persephone's Veil* and *Finding Love by Design*, designed to guide clients on their unique journeys of spiritual growth and relationship mastery. Connect with Icy on her website or follow her on social media to discover more about her life-changing offerings and insights.

You can connect with me on:

🌐 https://www.icykendrick.com

Subscribe to my newsletter:

✉ https://www.icykendrick.com

Also by Icy Kendrick

Explore My Other Works

Welcome, As you hold this book in your hands, I want you to know that you've stepped into a sacred space one where transformation, healing, and self-discovery unfold. This isn't just a collection of words; it's an invitation to journey deeper into yourself and the Spirit that flows through us all.

Each of my books was birthed with the intention of guiding you through life's most profound challenges and celebrating your divine power. Whether you're seeking clarity, healing, or a spark of inspiration, these works were designed to meet you exactly where you are and walk alongside you toward where you're destined to be.

These works aren't just books; they're experiences. They're my gift to you, born from the lessons I've learned, the battles I've fought, and the wisdom Spirit has poured into me.

So dive in, my dear. There's a book here calling your name, ready to ignite your fire, heal your wounds, and remind you of the magic within. Thank you for trusting me to walk this path with you.

With love and light,
   Icy The Medium Kendrick

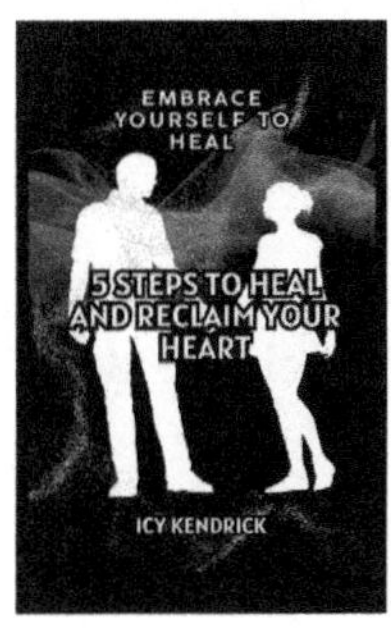

"5 Steps to Heal and Reclaim Your Heart"

https://www.icykendrick.com

This guide will hold your hand through heartbreak, showing you how to transform pain into a stepping stone for empowerment. It's a love letter to the parts of you that feel forgotten, reminding you that you are whole and worthy.

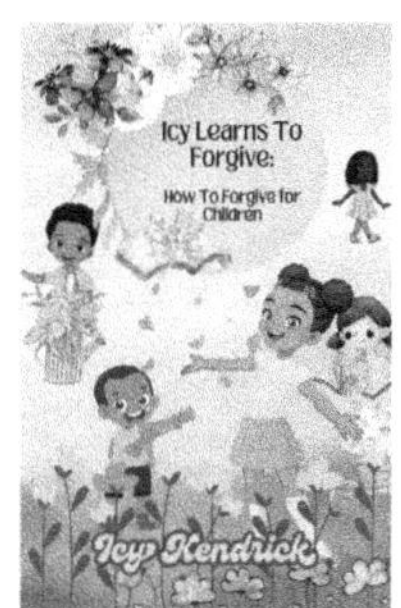

"Icy Learns to Forgive"

https://www.icykendrick.com

: A deeply personal tale inspired by my own journey, this book is a beacon for anyone learning to let go of resentment and open their heart to forgiveness.

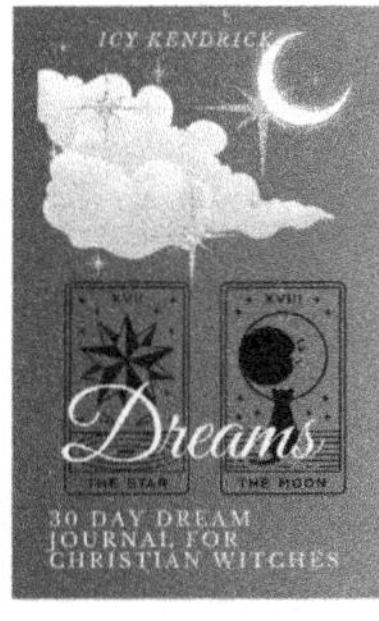

"30-Day Dream Journal for Christian Witches"

https://www.icykendrick.com

: Dreams are messages from the Spirit, whispering truths about your path. This journal is your sacred space to record, reflect, and decode the divine insights woven into your nights.

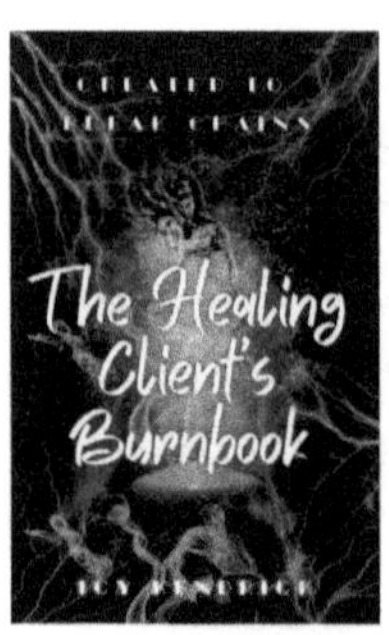

"The Healer's Client Burnbook: You Were Created to Break Chains"

https://www.icykendrick.com

: A fierce, unapologetic guide for healers to stand in their power and release what no longer serves them. This book is your permission slip to be bold, brave, and boundless.

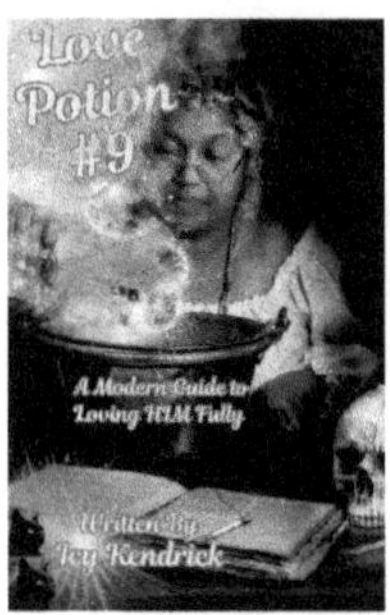

"Love Potion No. 9: A Modern Guide to Loving Him Fully"

https://www.icykendrick.com

: Whether you're in love or seeking it, this book is your blueprint for creating a connection that's both magical and real. A fresh, soulful perspective on navigating modern relationships.

www.ingramcontent.com/pod-product-compliance
Lightning Source LLC
Chambersburg PA
CBHW072337270726
48659CB00022B/1804